T0246505

Praise for *Good Grief*

"Brianna Pastor is by far one of my favorite new writers. *Good Grief* is a powerful testament that shows how hard the past can be and that overcoming it is possible. If you want to feel seen and deeply moved, read *Good Grief*. Brianna Pastor has unparalleled talent; let the power of her writing guide you to a better life."

—yung pueblo, #1 *New York Times* bestselling author

"If you're looking for raw, real, vulnerable truth, this collection is for you."

—Alexandra Elle, *New York Times* bestselling author of *How We Heal*

"Brianna Pastor's poetic debut does not disappoint and will resonate with many. *Good Grief* (amazing title!) is a poignant introductory collection that sets the stage beautifully for what's to come from Pastor."

—Alicia Cook, author of *Sorry I Haven't Texted You Back*

"When you read Brianna Pastor's words, it's like looking into a mirror. In *Good Grief,* she captures what many people ponder in silence. If you're looking for poetry and prose that soothe your soul, this book is for you."

—Terence Lester, founder of Love Beyond Walls and author of *I See You*

"*Good Grief* is emotional, raw, and powerful. It touches on emotions that often go unnoticed and unnamed. It touches on places that usually only the silence of the night knows. This book will have you cry and feel seen in ways you didn't even know you needed. I highly recommend you pick up a copy today."

—Christine Gutierrez, author of *I Am Diosa*

good grief

good grief

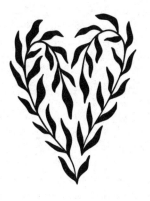

brianna pastor

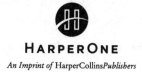

HARPERONE

An Imprint of HarperCollins*Publishers*

HarperCollins books may be purchased for educational, business, or sales promotional use. For information, please email the Special Markets Department at SPsales@harpercollins.com.

FIRST EDITION

Designed by Yvonne Chan
Floral illustrations © Yamurchik/Shutterstock

Library of Congress Cataloging-in-Publication Data has been applied for.

ISBN 978-0-06-335965-9

24 25 26 27 28 LBC 8 7 6 5 4

for the hurt, the healing, and everything in between

foreword

i started following brianna pastor's work about two years ago and was struck by her unique voice. she brought a different and much-needed tone to the topics of overcoming trauma, deep healing, and the transformation that occurs when an individual embraces their power. the way she brings together words makes the reader feel like developing a better life is genuinely possible.

we live in a special time when more people are turning inward to explore their conditioning and finding ways to unbind the past that causes them tension. brianna has arrived in the writing world at a critical moment; her work will continue pushing the movement of inner transformation forward.

i feel fortunate to have read her work and feel excited for those who are encountering her pieces for the first time. not only is her work inspiring but it also helps us slow down and truly feel, which is such a gift in a world that is often moving too fast. i hope her writing inspires you as deeply as it has inspired me.

yung pueblo, *new york times* bestselling author

author's note and trigger warning

i chose not to name these poems or put them in any particular order. if i name them, they stay with me, and i am more than ready to let them go. i put these poems out into the world as a releasing—a releasing of old patterns, traumas, and habits that i no longer wish to carry with me. while these poems will always be special to me, they were written during some of my lowest points. i will keep them there and go back to honor them when necessary. essentially, this book is a symbol of growth.

the contents in this book discuss topics such as mental health, depression, and trauma. *good grief* is a collection of poems and prose written over the last ten years—in my journey through both light and dark times. read along with me as i write to navigate my journey through self-worth and depression, identity, loss, and growth. i want this book to hold you warmly, as a reminder that you are never alone and that you are oh so capable. i wrote this for me but also very much for you.

thank you for being here and walking beside me.

good grief

the skin on my body healed itself in four days. that is how i knew that we are meant to overcome devastation, and that we complicate it by hanging on to what is no longer hurting us. we cling to pain like a parasite to its host.

with the proper care, i have avoided any infection. i was not going to allow further suffering for a small wound that burned so terribly in the moment.

we don't know how long our pain will last. we assume that because it hurts now, it is probably going to hurt tomorrow. it may even hurt the next day. perhaps it will get worse. but we sleep, you see, and we do this marvelous thing in our sleep—we mend.

and tomorrow is not always what we thought it would be.

not every apology
consists of words
you must feel it in your spine
the loosening of your posture
is synonymous with
forgiveness

when we hold on to resentment
the tower leans
and we don't see anything
for what it really is

the sun was my most-dreaded morning routine.
one aspect i could not change,
no matter how many attempts at
opaque curtains
i had draped over-top of each other.
it was hard to tell whether music made me feel sick
or if it reminded me of how happy i could have been
if only i had sung along
the way my sadness sang with the birds—
persistent, with purpose, and sharp.
there are distance runners that start in my chest,
down my arms and legs,
and for every mile they run
a coach tells them to make another round.
how do i get up and start the day
when there are people who run for miles
and i just run away

when water starts to boil,
it also begins to evaporate
don't let your anger boil so
intensely
that you start to lose sight of
who you are

there is no poem that will do
depression any justice—
for that gnawing feeling,
the creeping of its footsteps
emerging up the spiral staircase
i call my rib cage.

i think my mind wants to go to war, but
my body is
begging
for truce.

i opened my eyes, put two feet on the floor, began to walk, and my knees didn't give out. i walked to my kitchen, drank some coffee, looked out the window, and the sun burned my eyes. i allowed it. i walked over to the couch, sat down, turned on the television. i put on a show and didn't pay attention to it. i just wanted to feel like there were people around me. i sat blankly and stared around the room, trying to decide if i could move or if i needed to stay where i was. i have been frozen in time, lately. i always mourn in the morning. this is nothing new to me. but i want to know when the grief will shine through the window and enliven me. i want to know when my feet won't be nearly as heavy and when coffee won't taste like the day i didn't come visit you in the hospital. i want to know when being around actual people won't be as terrifying as it used to be. because now i know that if i'm around them, one day i could lose them, and i'll stay in this vicious cycle. all of this seems so far out of my reach. so for now, i'll lie in the bed as long as i need to. i'll listen to the faint noises of the house settling and drive myself crazy trying to find meaning in the silence. i'll find different ways to make my coffee and close my eyes when the sun hurts. i'll move softer so that i do not let this feeling go unfelt. because i loved you too much to not feel the weight of your absence.

today
i remember all of the selves i ever was
i forgive them for their self-inflicted pain
i commend them for their bravery and dignity
i sometimes miss them—in all their freeness
i ask myself now, if i am more afraid than i was back then—
and they answer:

fear lies beneath the layers
of which you will always uncover
but you will keep flying on.

the sea and i,
we stare at each other like distant relatives
who remember the pain they are bonded by

it will come for you.
through hell or high water
there is no need to dwell
or blame
or curse yourself
it is not your fault
if what you are chasing
wants your patience first

be careful what you
long for
because it just might
pass you by

a friend once described me as "flammable."
as soon as i heard the word from her mouth,
something inside of me blew apart.

it could mean many things.
but this is when i realized that it's just as
easy to set my soul on fire
as it is to watch me come crumbling down.

i return to ashes either way.

the thought of loving somebody
somebody's body
has grown into a new meaning for me.
because
i don't want somebody
to love my body
and leave it lonely.

trusting yourself is a
fiery thing
how freeing it is
to let life unfold
and still feel safe

i know that trauma lives in my body. i think it moved in and took reign over my house. i say this because i'm pretty sure that my teeth are sunken gravestones, and when i speak, i'm the only one around to listen.

your traumas
are never indicative of
who you are
and how well
you deserve to be loved

sometimes you walk,
and you won't get there in time.

sometimes you run,
and it has already passed you.

sometimes you get there
at exactly the right time,
at exactly the right speed,
and it still does not happen.

when it is for you,
it will be for you.

you are in every single thing you see. every single thing you touch. every life you pass through or step in. once your energy has been placed there, nothing is ever exactly the same as it was.

your brain remembers even the smallest of fragmented details about the places you have been and the way a person has reacted and the way a room feels when you enter or leave it.

leave everything with absolute love. your spirit matters beyond your own perception of it.

love does not equate to staying quiet.
sometimes
it has to be outspoken,
always loud,
and forever on fire.

i am growing backwards
a dark spiral into the opposite direction
and so different from everyone around me.
there are no branches for you to hang on to
just a simple me, an emotion tree
not growing for you to
grow off of or to destroy.

leave me be, so i may grow strong,
on my own,
and i will be my own damn home.

i came out of the womb crying,
like most people do—
except i just never stopped.

the truth is that there is no right answer. there is only what is right for you, what feels good to you, what you learn from each given situation, what you take away from every experience. when you spend too much time dwelling on answers you expect to be delivered to you, you miss opportunities to find them within yourself. you rob yourself of the chance to cultivate goodness for yourself. once we can learn to be so rooted in our entirety, this general acceptance feels a lot like cultivating a higher ground. a place where you can stand assured. a place where you can look below at the contents of your life and breathe.

it scared me. it scared me so much.
and that is why i had to do it.

there's about three feet of distance between my inner peace and my delicate romance with sadness. i'm afraid that if i mend that gap, there will be nothing left to measure here.

there are porch lights that stay on
and i always wonder who's inside
waiting—
and if their heart is hurting,
i hope the light is for them.

i step on the cracks anyway
because i know nothing in this life
could ever truly break my mother

letting go is actually the easiest decision we can make. we become so adapted to the weight of our heavy hearts that becoming *light* again is a foreign concept.

i know you squeeze into tight spaces
with the hope that you may fit
without aching.

there are spaces meant for you
that will not require you to bend
in order to belong safely.

it is safe to say that
nothing is safe
besides this moment
and yesterday.
that is why we touch it.

do not look me in the face.
my apologies
if my weak cheekbones offend you today;
i haven't quite been myself.
perhaps my bones have begun to
take the form of the pillow that
i have made my home.
or became concave from the incessant
inhalation of cigarette,
after cigarette,
after cigarette.
there is no beauty here.
no romance in my toxic solace.
i do not find comfort in the
excuses i spoon-feed you,
i cannot cover up my lethargy in
grandiose, theatrical performances
to spare you the
i don't know how to help her
or the
oh no not this again

i loved my sadness
because it was honest

you need both the light and the dark. one does not exist without the other. to sweep your darkness under the rug is to do yourself a great disservice. there is so much there to learn. how can you feel the freedom of the sun when you have not sat for a while under the shade of the trees? surely you can learn to appreciate both. the key here is learning to accept and exist in each state. to appreciate and welcome each part of you without discrediting it. we are creatures of light and dark. that is the space where strength and softness make a blood pact.

your split ends
and my split ends
are not the same.
my split ends suffer
immeasurable breakage
even after i trim them off,
and always
at the most desperate hours
of the night

i am alive to learn and unlearn, to relearn and unlearn and learn again. i am here to unpack and develop and understand the value in struggle. i am here to hold my grief the way it deserves to be held, for as long as that takes. i am here to learn that there is no judgment where there is love. i am here to understand that i am not small. i am here, and i am learning that this is a big thing.

i tend to resonate most
with people who
forget that they are loved
it's almost as if we forget that
we are living an experience
we get so caught up
in the world around us
that we forget
there is a worthy one within us
i feel the need to remind each of you
that you are loved
even if you feel lost
between both worlds

my boundaries are not
up for discussion or debate
they are clear, sturdy fences
and all of a sudden
you have the energy to jump them

i grow tired of your yearning excuses
and coincidentally, you love on me
when i don't need it to survive
anymore

you claim to have raised me to be
the strong one
when i find myself needing to be that
for myself, against you,

only then are you
kissing your teeth for it

i wrote delicate love notes to the earth / on my six-year-old, worn-out converse / in hopes that when i walked / she would hear my / incessant trying / an apology / to make up for / how heavy / my steps were / i hope that she understood / i hope that in her heart, she forgave me a couple of years back, i found the strength to ask one of my abusers how it felt to know that he had shoved my face so deeply into the mud that i am still pulling bits of soil from my teeth.

he told me that *i should have known better than to open my mouth*.

i give my sadness a full name
so that i stop thinking of her
as an intruder
and start acknowledging
that i do have to learn
how to live with her

you
catastrophically think
and i
catastrophically
tear my soul apart

—the first time i was ever truly seen

there is a constant duet in my head
one voice so soft, and one
an uproar:
both singing; reaching,
for some kind of peace;
and even on my most harmonious days,
i'm not sure that peace ever finds me.

i'm sorry
you cannot wake up
at the crack of dawn every morning
contemplating your best scheme
to make your amends with me

i have lain awake between
four cold, uptight walls
every night for twenty-seven years
contemplating my own worth
and existence because of you

if you ask me,
my burdens outspeak your guilt
actually, i don't know
your burden just might be
too much for me to ever carry
had it been my own

i am not sorry
for what you chose to do
or not do with your love

this body was my very own
first place of residence
it did not need fixing,
it needed to be appreciated
for the home it was

my body screams
please don't mind the mess,
i swear it's not always like this

my heart screams
come in
and love me regardless

i remember being five years old
and i remember the shadow
that never left me

where am i? why am i here?

every voice i heard was strung
in hatred, in misery, in shielded fear
carved, now, onto the insides of my skin

your words.
you didn't hear yourself
when you were speaking—
your anger created
a poorly written song
with a catchy tune
the song that always seems
to be stuck in my head
and crawls back to me out of the blue

and when times are fearful,
i can even dance to it

"no" is also an action
let it be your own approval
of disapproval
wear it around your neck
as you lift your chin to turn away
even if your skin feels different
even if "yes" tries to follow
up the back of your throat

i take great comfort in knowing
there are even better versions of myself
that i haven't hugged yet

i want to love the universe the way it has not loved me

just because you called out my name
and i did not speak
does not mean that i was absent
we are not children in a classroom
i do exist
without your acknowledgment
i am here
even if you do not see me

you broke my heart so many times
i spent so many years after you
trying to find a bond
without the defeat
only to learn that the bond
was a leash

and then there was six-year-old me
dishing out cries in acronyms with sharpie marker
across my wooden bunk bed:

IHTW
IHTW
IHTW

my mother questioned why
i hate the world
when i hadn't even slightly touched it yet

my only explanation
is that i hated the parts i had already seen—
why would i want to see more?

for a very long time
i disgusted myself
because i didn't say yes
but i didn't say no.

i thought,
is this what love feels like?
and then learned that it wasn't.

you told me not to chew on bottle caps
because you didn't want me to ruin my teeth
but you had no problem with watching me love
people who were no good to me

one night i found myself stumbling into my regular coffee shop to write. it was my safe space. i sat down in front of a napkin that someone had left behind. it read, "un jour, je découvrirai le secret pour que mes yeux soient moins lourds. ils ne guérissent jamais des pleurs."

i took out my phone to translate: "one day i will discover the secret to having my eyes feel less heavy. they never heal from the crying."

i sat in place and silently mourned. not only did i find the answer to why i kept ending up in this coffee shop alone, but i also felt empathy for a world that is sad *in so many different languages.*

i need you to meet me in the room
where identity meets safety
the room where we gather—
to learn what this feels like
so that we can replicate this same room
within ourselves

i never know what to say when people ask me about myself. i have never been good at letting someone know me before i have the chance to worry about them knowing me. maybe that is a bad thing. maybe i know that i'm more than they could handle. maybe i know that not many people can appreciate somebody whose peace comes with a somber aftertaste. maybe i don't know the simple way to tell them that i'm the person who dreams during the day and gets one or two layers thinner at night. sometimes three. have you ever met a person who walks slower next to the man in the wheelchair on the sidewalk because she feels sick to her stomach that she might make him sad? i haven't—i just know that i am more than what others want to expect of me. that they might look at my heavy face and try to read it like hieroglyphics. and i know that they probably wouldn't understand.

i dread the day these demons come back for me
they have gone away to pursue better things
but can never find what they're looking for
so here they come, back to me,
a place where they are not wanted—
for they always stop by unannounced
and don't understand the concept of *manners*
in another person's home

there will be no more
spreading myself thin
across my bedroom floor
to have everything
covered at once

i have split myself down
into enough layers
to cover this floor like tile
for nine of my lifetimes

i swear the entire sky was on fire when you died
i thought:
this is how she would leave the world
i can't think of a better way for her to be
here and there and everywhere else
she can see the entire world from above
before she leaves it
better than it had ever left her

i'll be damned.
you really were too good for
what you were given

there is nowhere to run to
and so much to run from
i study so much about
the process of trust
but i am literal enough to know
you cannot trust a single, tangible thing
not with anything important, anyway
and everything big and small
is best kept between my two ears
and swarming around my chest
and twitching in my legs
and buzzing at my fingertips
and crying in italicized letters

i put my Grief in the corner
between the dusty nightstand and
a pile of clean laundry
Grief concentrates on the line that separates each wall
and how many accidental scratches she can find to pass the time
and her legs wobble after the first two hours
Grief eventually does grow tired
despite her consistency
don't turn around
dissociate instead
she closes her eyes and stretches
leans her head against the corner
Grief asks if she is allowed to have dinner but
you don't feed Grief
Grief feeds you

i don't think that i had much of a choice
when my Grief and i became one entity
so i learned to sleep
i learned it was the only way for me to leave

it is said that the cells of me once existed
in the bellies of my ancestors
that i was predestined to be here
before i was ever an ounce of a thought
if these insecure legs
and rigid elbows existed
long before i hated them,
perhaps i should give them a chance
to be as beautiful as their origin

anxiety
holds me tight around the knees
like a begging child
waiting for me to give in
to whatever it is that he wants.

they tell you to learn discipline.
they tell you that if you give in,
he will never learn.
if you don't hold your head up strong,
he will grow not to know
any better.

you become so tired of the hounding,
the nagging screech coming from below,
that you figure:
it will be easier if i just give him what he wants.
if i just
yes him to death
maybe the noise will subside.

until you are in the supermarket
with your mother,
for the first time in what feels like
your entire life.
out of almost thin air, to your surprise,
the child is back around your knees.
crying, taunting, begging for dear life
that you'll give in once more and
he will continue to return until you do because
he only knows how to go home
and you have already created a home within you.

good grief, you are lazy. that's what she always tells me. you spend so much time asleep that you can't possibly still be tired. that's what you think. little did she know that in my dreams, i ran around town trying to salvage what is left of me. i searched far and wide for something to rescue me. to put an end to me. be a friend to me. *good grief.* she says i have too much time to think. i don't know what more she expects from me. i was made to have this body but this body keeps rejecting me. *good grief.* she says she doesn't know how to help me. for once i can say that we don't disagree. i wish you could have been my eyes when i couldn't see. this wasn't something i could pretend to be. depression took everything away from me. *good grief.*

do you fear me? love asked.
no.
i fear that of which inhibits you.

1. maybe if i number what i am trying to tell you, you will take it as something you need to get done
2. you have always been good at making lists for yourself
3. i need you to know that i have never felt like my life has mattered to you
4. your form of nurture only consists of asking me mundane things at the end of the day and suggesting i call my doctor
5. almost nobody i know is ever a healthy body with a constant headache
6. i list things out for you but mostly for myself
7. the numbers remind me that there have been too many cries and not enough breakthroughs

abandoned tree trunks sprawl out across the dilapidated yard,
remnants from last year's party are still down by the river
i sit up from bed at five in the afternoon and light my cigarette.
i have already missed the daylight
sweet, sweet daylight, i hate you
people live during the day and become who
they are at night
i see a yellow-lit window off in the distance
every night i watch the person in the room
dance ballet in their robe
and leave for work in the morning in a fancy suit
i want to know who you are in front of the moon
i want to know who you are when you have
nobody
and only your heart

a month ago to this day, i turned thirty. i never envisioned this happening. when i was nine, i thought i knew everything there was to know about the world. i thought that to be thirty was to see more of the same despair and i didn't think that was something to look forward to. you may know me at thirty now. but you must first know me at nine. skin and bones, fear and tears, shame for being alive. a burden to walk. a burden to feel. a burden to every life i touched. you must know me at nineteen, when i had nowhere to go and a new truth when i understood that i was gay. you must know me at twenty-four, when i lived in a place where i washed my dishes in the bathtub because i couldn't afford a place with a kitchen. you must know how many times i had to put the dishes down, to cry into the floorboard. you must know how quiet that was from my chest. you must know me at thirty, what it has taken to get here. what has been taken from me, to get here. you must know that i awaken every day and fight through the trenches of absolute hell to keep going. it has been one month since i turned thirty. and because i never envisioned this, it means that maybe i get to create it. maybe i get to create a different story to tell thirty years later. and that is something i can envision now.

and if nothing else, please,
let your love be bigger
than your anger

there is no magic answer for how i ended up in a better place. but i can tell you how hard i pushed to get here. i started to pay attention to the way i greeted people, how i interacted with them on a daily basis. i started paying attention to the way others treated me. i started making sure the questions i brought to the table meant something. making sure they weren't empty. accompanying my smile with my eyes. having heart for others even when mine was hurting. i read a lot of books. and i mean, a lot of books. i wanted to learn about myself through something outside of myself. i read things i didn't fully understand so that there was room for interpretation. i became quiet and started watching those around me. i became quiet and i started to listen. pretending that i couldn't hurt enough for me to not listen to others. realizing that it was my choice to make: loving others despite personal circumstances.

i lost a lot of people in many different ways. i suffered deeply for those losses. i would be lying if i said that some of those losses weren't because i was struggling mentally. i asked myself important questions. what do i value? what kind of person would i be most proud of being? what do i enjoy? i found that community was important to me because i never had it. i learned to answer my questions. at the end of the day, everything came back to the importance of love. proving to myself that this love also included more of it for my own being. that without that, my love for others wouldn't be as whole as i intended for it to be. i wanted to make the most of my ability to love, so i began with myself. every day. even if i didn't fully understand what that looked like. regardless of how difficult it was to learn.

if anyone is magically going to appear
and suddenly make your life better,
just know that person
is always going to be you

there are people waiting to meet you.
people waiting to love you.
there are places that stand still
until you've stepped foot in them.
something really beautiful
could happen for you in the morning.
there is so much waiting for your arrival.
arrive there.

what you don't think about when you are stuck in a pattern is how fluid your thoughts are. we tend to grab on to thoughts as if we are running around catching fireflies in the dark. what we forget is that they are meant to exist and fly and carry on. our thoughts are just as transient. we must allow them to flow without feeling as though we must cage them and be caged *by* them.

i spend a generous amount of time
trying to convince myself that
i am worthy of taking up space
in a world that i find myself
constantly needing space from

and who will advocate for me?
me.
even when it feels lonely.
lonely is where i grow the most.

your growth will be more apparent
when it is being tested

on days when everything
feels like too much,
you are not abnormal

what is abnormal
is denying yourself the compassion
you would give so freely to others

you know what i did? i said "okay." i can feel this sadness and allow these thoughts today, but i won't let them stop me. so i acknowledged these thoughts and how they made me feel—i said them aloud. myself and i had a wonderful discussion about how i need to be softer. so i whispered, "okay, feel it, but we're not going to sit in it." and the more i talk with myself, the easier it is to lift myself out of my anguish. i kept going. i said "okay" to my uneasy feelings.

stare hard at the hurt
ask why it stings
dig into the root and rip it out
it does not have to stay there
just because it grew there

i am hell-bent
on loving my
hell

loneliness can be opportune for
learning radical acceptance
of your core self

it can be disguised as sadness
when you are not at ease with
who that may be

please do not rush my recovery
i am in a whirlpool of
"should be," "could be," "would be,"
when all i need is to
"be"

to heal is to turn yourself inside out to make amends

i know that i am terrified of loss. as if it could end me. as if it almost has. i live on the idea that things can stay "okay" within myself if we could freeze the "okay" moments. but the truth about moments is that they are fleeting, so fast that perhaps they aren't real. like this moment, right now: it is so far past us already that i figure, well, maybe we should just stay in this one. we are losing moments as we speak, without realizing that they are not tangible. even when they deeply touch us. loss is flowing. this moment is all we have, really. and i want to love it, even if i lose it.

my heart will follow your heart to all ends of the earth / like
a competitive game of musical chairs / like the flame of a
candle to oxygen / like a hopeful family to a missing child /
i will never give up on you / our souls overlap like a Venn
diagram / we have been finding each other in circles for the
last several lifetimes / i'm not letting you get away in this one

when i tell you that
i love you differently
than i have ever loved—

what i mean is that
i love you
and myself
at the same time

i don't want to
grow a thick skin

i want my skin
to stay
as thin as it was made
and
everything outside of that

to be softer

unconditional love
lets you cry flowers

it is the dark of winter
but i see gardens:
alive and well,
and thriving

learning how to love myself
has been a growing upward
and outward
and always
and a forever
please

i have gone to sleep sad so many times
i'm surprised i haven't woken up invisible yet

you had your "upper hand"
jammed so far down my throat
that i was so focused on
how i was going to breathe and
forgot that i had hands of my own
to stop you

pick it up. let it rest beside you. then, let it be.

i know that you have loved me to the
capacity at which you know how to.

i love you for that.

my mind became a castle in the sky
fusing together events i know
could never happen
afloat in the ocean
a body of a much bigger form than my own
that of which i am not accustomed to coping against.

but, i manage
and i lie there, with no worry in the world
of who i may be
or who i may not
what i can solidly remember and
the pain i thought i forgot.

the crisp severity of the ocean
on the outer layers of my skin
a rivalry—counteracting the heat
my anger is ceaselessly producing
an effortless breath of cold air
and no endurance needed to fight against the current
my head being totally consumed by waves,
in intervals but enough to refresh my inner cognition.

one deep inhale and i can feel you,
just before i start to slowly fade under,
and when i think this can't get any better,
i finally hear it. the thunder.
it's loud, and i've been waiting, and i am scared
but not worried enough to budge.
the storm is growing strong above my
physical, still body
and with the moving body below me
that i want to love so much.

what i can't grasp fully, though,
is the way i refuse to move
i know i am terrified of the consequences,

i'm already worrying
as i have been, this entire time
time figures out that it's not my body
that refuses to move
it is manipulated by my mind.

i am content here.
if i stay in this *opposing body*
it reminds me of all the things i do not have
rather than the things i do,
and can't accept.

i am saddened,
that my breaths were not voluntary
they were forced by the love i cannot feel.
i know it's there, i know it's real.
reminded by this ocean, i am very much alive.

and although inside i may feel broken and numb,
sometimes, i can be fine.

i remember
i think i always will

even as a child time always stood still

i want to forget—what a concept.
are we meant to remember?

i think i'm meant to remember.

so long as judgment exists—
nothing truly peaceful can thrive

i don't really understand
what surface level means

but i know that each emotion
i have ever felt
has never met any layer of my skin
before moving into
the marrow in my bones

if only we spoke in the language
of shapes and colors
maybe then
we would speak of love
like it was endearing

sometimes words
do their own damage
despite their intention

my mom didn't like to cook. i can't necessarily say that i blame her. often, we spent nights eating at a restaurant. i can't say that this was memorable, but i always looked forward to the car ride home. in the back of my mom's camaro, i'd lie down just enough to where i could see the moon. i wasn't old enough to understand that it wasn't following us home; the car was just moving. i always saw its face. the darker eyes and the subtle smirk. a face that promised rescue, a face that knew something i didn't yet.

just so you know—
i will never forget,
not for as long as i live.

i know you didn't love me,
but i really thought that you did

your softness never goes to waste

i think that i am much too anxious
to ever personally meet death.
i cannot see the day when
something so determined
is finally put in its place.

for death may say: *it is time*
but surely i would find a way
to think myself out of it.

you are not weak—
you are *hurting*

i have never seen a weak thing
change shape the way you do

crawl and shrivel and beg and adjust
just to make it to the next moment

i call this survival

there is a difference between
moving on and
forgetting

for example,
i have moved on from what you've done to me
but
i will never forget it

the thing is
when you're here
i don't know where to put you
you're either a part of me
or none of me
because i don't know where else
you're supposed to go
or how i'm supposed to make you
any smaller

i don't know how to compartmentalize love
or how to make the way you matter to me
less than
what i mean to myself

in totality,
i am more love
than i am
wound

more ease
than i am
hurry

more grounded
than i am
sky

i am not a girl or a boy / i do not want one career more than
the other / i don't want my depression to depend on my
time spent in the sun / i don't want my weight to be a scale i
base my worth upon / i don't want rain or shine / i want the
freeness that my body feels when no one else is near / i want
to wake up in the morning and choose my name, never the
same name twice / i want to dance and feel in total awe of
my bravery / i don't want to feel brave for being willing to
dance / i want people to think i've gone mad and laugh from
my belly about it / i want to be queer and define what that
means to me and not be banned for it / i want what life
was meant to be and not the cage it has become

i thought that "letting go" meant that i had to disregard a part of me that loved deeply. i thought that by learning to let go, i would no longer be able to protect myself or those i love. trauma has made me correlate a fear of losing control to who i am as a person. a person who does not let go. i allowed myself to identify with fear and used it as a personality trait to defend my devotion to others. this is not love, and this is not who i am. sometimes love requires "letting go" in the sense that we must abandon need for control. love flows easier when there is no grip on it.

the face you see here
resembles a bare land mine:
sensitive, urgent, waiting.
i have known the pain
of waiting all my life—
for exploding when
others step on me and
the dust that lingers on for miles.
i am both the land mine and
the one who steps on it
i am the one who grieves the loss
and carries the guilt
and i also want you to know
that part of me will always be active
but there is a much less dangerous one
here now, and ahead—

i have grown, tremendously,
like rapid fire.
i am no longer explosive
in the way that i once was.
i am learning that there are
better ways
to make a big deal of me.

i want to apologize to myself
for constantly submerging in
a state of panic

for allowing myself to
self-destruct
for so many years

there is a person inside of me
who deserves kindness

i didn't know what to do
so i did nothing
and in doing nothing
i then understood
what needed to be done

what is this radical idea that we are different?
we are the same, you and i

we come, we feel, and we go

see.
think.
think again.
love.

sometimes, i consider myself
to be the wind

sometimes, i consider myself
to be the anchor

sometimes, i know that without a doubt,
i am the ocean

but only the open sky can see
what i really am

and so, we meet here, in the place
between everything light and dark
there will always be safety here for you
because i have created it for me
and for all the intricate versions of ourselves
that we will ever be